YOUR KNOWLEDGE HAS VALUE

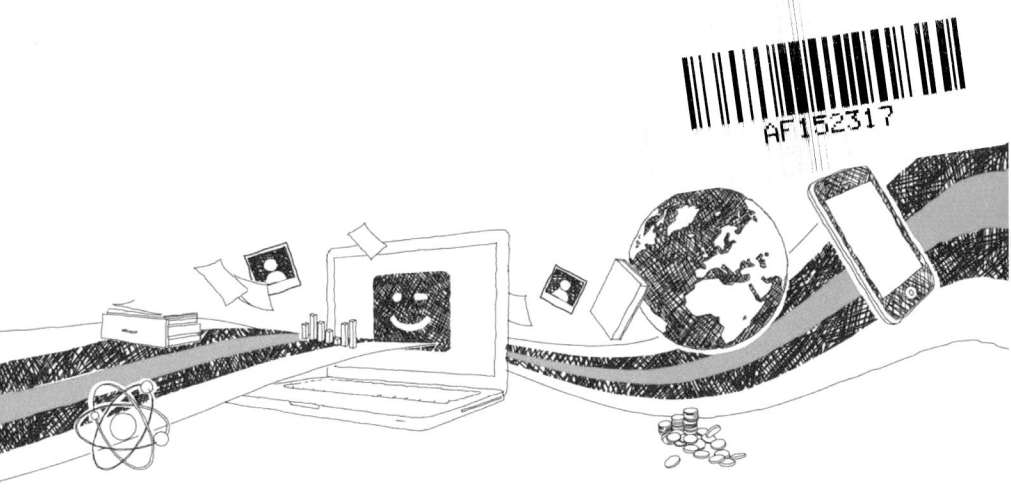
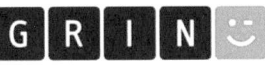

Yashveer Sachdev

Tuberculosis in Kenya

GRIN Publishing

Imprint:

Copyright © 2012 GRIN Verlag GmbH
Print and binding: Books on Demand GmbH, Norderstedt Germany
ISBN: 978-3-656-92565-1

This book at GRIN:

http://www.grin.com/en/e-book/294398/tuberculosis-in-kenya

GRIN - Your knowledge has value

Since its foundation in 1998, GRIN has specialized in publishing academic texts by students, college teachers and other academics as e-book and printed book. The website www.grin.com is an ideal platform for presenting term papers, final papers, scientific essays, dissertations and specialist books.

The Republic of Kenya is a third world country located in East Africa and has a number of issues (health and otherwise). Kenya is poor in terms of its economics; it is a low income developing country where agriculture sustains 80% of the people; relying on maize as its chief food crop and coffee and tea as the main cash crops (Kenya 2008). Kenya's multiparty democracy and strong central government allows healthcare officials and researchers to communicate with them. However, Kenya has trouble providing adequate healthcare for its population. One of the health issues that Kenya must concern itself with is Tuberculosis and this can present itself with other medical conditions as well, such as HIV.

Tuberculosis infected 9.4 million patients in 2009 and nearly 14 million people are living with the disease worldwide. Kenya is one of the 22 World Health Organization defined high burden countries where 80% of the world's burden for TB exists; it is 13th amongst the 22 high burden Tb countries (Billingsley et al. 2008). Tb is underreported; furthermore, Tb-related morbidity, mortality and drug resistance are expected to increase (Ayisi, Hoo, Agaya, Mchombre, Nyamthimba, Muhenje and Marstonn 2011). The Estimated number of new Tb cases in Kenya is around 130,000 (Infectious Diseases, Kenya, 2009). Estimated Tb prevalence in Kenya is around 300/100,000 (Infectious Diseases, Kenya, 2009). From 2006 to 2009, the total number of newly registered Tuberculosis patients reported each year decreased 5% from 115,234 to 110,015. Kenya has experienced an increase in TB detection rates from 51 to 320 per 100,000 between 1987 and 2004 (Billingsley et al. 2008). The Tb case detection rate is the number of incident TB cases in a given year (Mansoer, Schecle, Floyd, Dye, Sitiene, and Williams 2009).

Tuberculosis is caused by the bacterium Mycobacterium Tuberculosis (Basic TB Facts 2012). Mycobacterium Tuberculosis usually attacks the lungs, but it can also attack the kidneys, spine and brain. Tb is spread via air contact/droplets; person with Tb can spread it by coughing, sneezing or speaking; it is not spread by touch (Basic TB Facts 2012).

In order to formulate a plan to deal with Tuberculosis in Kenya, I followed what was done in the past. The plan would be to learn as much about the disease process and the disease in Kenya first and then figuring out what resources are needed (partially by contacting organizations) and partly by looking at previous research. Then it would be necessary to diagnose the disease, educate the public and actually treat cases of the disease, paying attention to any health, social and political repercussions.

The first step would be gathering information and knowledge of the disease in certain regions of Kenya. It would be important to know what information can be gathered and which cannot and how to go about gathering that knowledge. Electronic databases can be used to gather this information.

The next step would be figuring out what resources (monetary and otherwise) would be necessary to treat and prevent Tuberculosis. There are multiple sources of care available for Tuberculosis and there are also problems with access and affordability (Ayisi et al. 2011). There are private facilities that charge fees for service, but they were not selected; the focus here is on the public sector (Mauch et al. 2011). Issues to be considered with having public facilities active and available are costs for diagnostic tests and costs for treatment, administrative charges (personnelle need to be hired), medicines taken for TB symptoms, transport to and from health facilities, food and supplements and accommodation costs (Mauch et al. 2011).

After that it would be necessary to educate the public. One of the issues related to Tb is that patients are unsure about the causes of Tb; some examples of what Kenyans thought caused Tb are alcohol, certain drinking water, sharing utensils and physical labor (Ayisi et al. 2011). Education is necessary to dispel myths and spread knowledge about Tb, but it should be noted that popular and folk beliefs of the patients are mixed in as well and there are "therapeutic narratives" where people assign person and social meaning to illnesses; the health beliefs may come from the professional health sector, popular sector or social sector (family and friends) (Ayisi et al. 2011).

The public should be diagnosed and we should understand the disease ramifications. It is difficult to measure the incident of TB disease directly. Significant progress has been made in TB control over the last 10 years and again it is often studied with concurrent infections; almost all patients are also tested for HIV (Mansoer et al. 2009).

There is a social stigma associated with Tb even though patients in Kenya have reported that those around them did not treat them differently. Defaulting from treatment is also a problem because there is a lack of knowledge/misconception about the duration of Tb treatment; patients have stopped taking the treatments because they felt the treatments lasted too long (Ayisi et al. 2011).

After that, the next step would be to test and treat the public. A patient should get tested for Tb if they are or have been 1) exposed to Tb patients, 2) Immunocompromised, 3) show signs and symptoms of Tb or 4) use illegal drugs. A full diagnosis of Tb is made via a) Medical History, b) Physical Exam, c) Tb injection test, d) Chest radiograph and e) Lab tests . 2 kinds of tests are used: TB skin test (TST) and TB blood tests (Testing for TB Infection 2011). A positive test indicates that a person has been infected; it does not indicate whether the person has latent TB infection or has progressed to TB disease. The TB skin test is the Mantoux skin test in which a small amount of fluid (called Tuberculin) is injected into the skin into the larger part of the arm (Testing for TB Infection 2011). Tb blood tests measure how the immune system reacts to the bacteria that cause Tb.

2

It should be noted that many of the participants delayed seeking treatment for various reasons, in one study for example, the majority of participants felt that their symptoms were not serious enough and patients also often use self-treatment before going to see a healthcare provider (Ayisi et al. 2011).

Lastly, we must prevent the disease or reduce future Tb outbreaks. BCG is the vaccine for Tb; it is seen in persons born outside the United States, but it can interfere with test results and give a false positive (Testing for TB Infection 2011). Since the economically vulnerable are more likely to contract Tb, the previously mentioned economic constraints must be considered. A "Medical Poverty Trap" exists that can spiral a patient into deeper poverty. The inability to work is a major cause of increased poverty and contributes to worsening of individual economic situations; potential income that is lost to TB is entered as a cost as well (Mauch et al. 2011). The indirect costs of the entire duration of illness constituted 85% of total costs and most patients had to borrow money or sell assets to cover costs incurred (Mauch et al. 2011).

In order to implement the ideas listed in the planning process, it is first and foremost necessary to communicate with organizations that are based/located in, have worked in or have contact with Kenyan authorities, the Kenyan government and Kenyans. They should understand the nature of the environment and would be able to direct me as to which course of actions to take. Technology and tools that have already been developed can be used to help facilitate this whole process.

TB patients have a substantial burden of direct (out of pocket) and indirect costs due to TB (Mauch et al. 2011). These economic burdens were measured and tracked using a mathematical and statistics tool created in Kenya to help control programs. The tool created also assesses previous TB treatment episodes, health seeking behaviors and delays and costs to the supporter of the patient. The tool was piloted in Kenya where TB diagnosis and treatment at public facilities were free of charge (Mauch et al. 2011). Not only was the assessment tool used, but a questionnaire was provided as well; this questionnaire was translated into Kiswahili and back translated into English (Mauch et al. 2011).

Well known organizations that should be contacted are The Centers for Disease Control, DLTLD and The Health and Demographic Surveillance System (HDSS) in Western Kenya and the Kenyan National Tuberculosis control program which follows the internationally recommended DOTS program (Mauch et al.2011). DOTS is the World Health Organization's strategy vs. Tb. Kenya began the DOTS program in 1993 and met the target goal of 85% by 2007 (Infectious Diseases, Kenya, 2009). DLTLD is Kenya's national division of Leprosy, TB and Lung disease and is responsible for overseeing clinical activities at around 2200 Tb diagnostic and treatment facilities (Mansoer et al. 2009). Furthermore, ethical clearance needs to be provided; for example, in one study it was done by the Kenyan medical

Research Institute (KEMRI) and the Centers for Disease Control and Prevention (CDC) In Atlanta, Georgia (Ayisi et al.2011).

US AID provided $2.9 million in 2008 to Kenya to help fight Tb and recommends that there should be 1) utilization of software (Epi Info 6.0 is an example), 2) there should be better nationwide DOTS coverage, 3) new lab equipment should be used, 4) there should be increased communication and we should 5) work with companies to promote Tb awareness (Infectious Diseases, Kenya, 2009).

In order to adequately treat Tb as part of the plan, there should be 1) standard screening procedures, 2) additional training of healthcare workers, 3) additional education of patients, 4) better access to diagnostic tests, 5) reduced costs of diagnostic tests and 6) better communication with patients (low knowledge of Tb and low suspicion of the disease among the staff is a concern (Ayisi et al. 2011).

After all actions are performed in and on behalf of healthcare in Kenya, an evaluation must be performed to see if any of the results were positive. This information will help any future researchers and healthcare workers planning to work in that area, will help reduce the plans and patterns that not strategically sound and hopefully this information can be contribute to some official database, partially so that the work and efforts can be reflected upon. Retrospective chart reviews have been used for data collection in quality assessment and improvement work (Billingsley et al. 2008). A data extraction tool for retrospective chart review based on the International Standards for TB Care can be used in settings where resources are limited. Tools such as these are field tested at specific locations, but need to be tested at other sites and also in non-specific broad areas (Billingsley et al. 2008). Chart reviews and data collection can be again entered into computer programs such as excel and SPSS. Retrospective chart reviews are common in quality improvement literature, but have limitations in that the recorded data may be inaccurate or incomplete (Billingsley et al.2008). Throughout the process, if this information was to be used for research purposes, it is important to remember that Informed consent must be provided and interviews must conducted by trained staff in private rooms and should cover the topics of 1) symptom onset, 2) perceived cause, 3) how treatment was sought and how long it took to get that care. Convenience sampling, rather than random sampling is recommended because it has the advantage of easily identifying patients (Ayisi et al. 2011).

References

Ayisi, J.G., Hoo, A.H., Agaya, J.A., Mchombre, W., Nyamthimba, P.O., Muhenje, O. and Marston, B.J. (2011). Care Seeking and Attitudes towards treatment compliance by newly enrolled tuberculosis patients in the district treatment programme in rural western Kenya; a qualitative study. BMC Public Health, 11:515, 1-10.

Basic TB facts. (2012). Centers for Disease Control and Prevention. Retrieved from www.cdc.gov/tb/topic/basics/default.htm#

Billingsley, K. M., Smith, N., Shirley, R., Achieng, L. and Keiser, P.(2011). A quality assessment tool for tuberculosis control activities in resource limited settings. *Tuberculosis, 91*, 549-553.

Infectious Diseases, Kenya (2009). USAID. Retrieved from www.cdc.gov/our_work/global_health/id/tuberculosis/countries/africa/kenya_profile.html

Kenya. (2008). In Philip's Encyclopedia 2008. Retrieved from http://ezproxy.shu.edu//login?qurl=http%3A%2F%2Fwww.credoreference.com/entry/philipency/kenya

Mansoer, J., Schecle, S., Floyd, K., Dye, C., Sitiene, J., and Williams, B. (2009). New Methods for estimating the tuberculosis case detection rate in high-HIV prevalence countries; the example of Kenya. Bull World Health Organ, 87, 186-192.

Mauch, V., Woods, N., Kirubi, B., Kirpruto, H., Sitiene, J., and Klinkenberg, E. (2011). Assessing access barriers to Tuberculosis care with the tool to Estimate Patient's costs; pilot results from two districts in Kenya. BMC Public Health, 11:43, 1-10.

Testing for TB infection (2011). Centers for Disease Control and Prevention. Retrieved from www.cdc.gov/tb/topics/testing/default.htm

Treatment. (2011). Centers for Disease Control and Prevention. Retrieved from www.cdc.gov/tb/topic/treatment/default.htm.